CANCER:
A CHRISTIAN'S GUIDE TO
COPING
AND
CARING

CANCER:
A CHRISTIAN'S GUIDE TO
COPING
AND
CARING

Christine Blazer Bigley

Beacon Hill Press of Kansas City
Kansas City, Missouri

10   9   8   7   6   5   4   3   2   1

Although a great many persons made this project possible, I want to dedicate this book to the special persons in the pilot support group at First Church of the Nazarene in Topeka, Kans.:

Ada
Audrey
Donavene
Ellamae
Esther
Marie
Maryeva
Rosella
Ruby
Ruth

CONTENTS

Foreword 9

Introduction 12

Part I

What You Need to Know About People and Cancer

1. What Cancer Victims Wish You Knew 19
2. Four More Things Cancer Victims
   Wish You Knew 27
3. What Family Members of Cancer Victims
   Wish You Knew 36
4. What Friends and Acquaintances
   of Cancer Victims Want to Know 41

Part II

What You Need to Know About the Christian Faith

5. What You Need to Know About
   God and Suffering 47
6. What You Need to Know About
   the Faith Community 58

Part III

What You Need to Know to Start a Support Group
for Cancer Victims in Your Church

7. How to Get Started..67
8. How to Use This Book as a Guide for a Support
   Group in Your Church 81

Epilogue 85

Notes 86

Bibliography 88

FOREWORD

How many people are in the room as you read this? Just you, your spouse, and the guy on the TV screen giving the weather report? That's three. The statistical probabilities are that one of you three will have cancer sooner or later—and you can't always count on it being the weatherman.

The incidence of cancer is on the rise. Who will offer personal and spiritual care to the millions of victims? Christine Bigley points out that both the suffering of victims and the example of our Lord Jesus Christ call us to minister to those lonely millions stricken by cancer.

A lot of people would like to help but don't know what to say or do. Dr. Bigley will help remedy that situation. In this book, she brings together the resources of the Christian faith and the tried and proven principles of clinical practice in the support of cancer victims. She believes and teaches that one does not have to be a medical or psychological professional to lead ministries to victims of cancer. Laypersons who are concerned about people can bring the resources of the community of faith to those suffering from cancer.

To be sure, the medical community is doing its part in advancing cancer treatment. A number of community service agencies are working to support cancer victims, their friends, and their families. But the government and community support groups are not permitted, in this pluralistic society of ours, to make the Christian faith a part of their service. That is one reason the Church must catch up with the medical and social service agencies. We have an essential and unique contribution to make.

The Church indeed sees suffering as more than pain and grief. Bound up in the mystery of suffering are nuances of redemptive value and real meaning. After all, when God decided to redeem the world, He chose to do it through suffering. We followers of His, who are, according to the Scriptures, commanded to "share" and to "complete . . . Christ's sufferings" (Col. 1:24, TEV), do not believe that suffering is wasted. Although we cannot explain it, we know that in some way our suffering, dedicated to God, works toward the ultimate redemption of the whole creation, which, as Paul says, groans as it awaits the day of redemption (Rom. 8:21-22).

Dr. Bigley is uniquely qualified to coach us on such matters. She is an unusual package of gifts and graces, education, and experience. She is a registered nurse and has served as a teacher of nurses. She is also trained as a minister of the gospel, holding M.Div. and D.Min. degrees from Nazarene Theological Seminary, Kansas City. She has served in parish ministry along with her husband, George. Further, she has logged nearly a decade of experience as a hospital chaplain. The program of ministry to cancer victims in the parish, which she proposes in this book, has been put to the test in actual parish work.

I had the privilege of looking over Dr. Bigley's shoulder as coach and encourager while she prepared this manuscript. I also had a chance to observe her in action. I visited a parish support group she was leading on a balmy June evening in Topeka, Kans.

The night I visited, Dr. Bigley adjourned the classroom part of the meeting early. She then loaded the whole group into one person's van and took them to a nearby hospital. You see, one member of the group was facing cancer surgery the next day. I watched with deep appreciation as the patient visited with eight other persons who really knew how Donavene felt.

It was a moment long to be remembered when eight cancer victims joined hands with the cancer-stricken patient in a prayer circle. Almost every member of the group led in prayer. It was an awesome moment.

If this book helps just one reader bring the kind of support that Donavene received from the group that night, I'm sure Dr. Bigley will feel that the hours, days, weeks, and months of sorting data, arranging information, writing, and rewriting will have been worth it.

WESLEY TRACY
Editor, *Herald of Holiness*
Kansas City

INTRODUCTION

You Are Not Alone

The fact that you are reading this page probably means that cancer has come close to you—perhaps invading your circle of friends, your family, or your own body.

You are not alone. Eighty-three million Americans now living will get cancer—about one in three. Three out of four families will be affected by the disease. The annual number of new cases, not including skin cancers, is 1.13 million. Over 8 million Americans alive today have a history of cancer, 4 million diagnosed five or more years ago.

Currently some 1,400 persons die of cancer each day, 520,000 annually. Lung cancer will claim 158,000 (most of these cases are related to tobacco smoke). One of every nine women you meet will sooner or later become a victim of breast cancer. If a family history of breast cancer exists, the risk is one in four. Men also get breast cancer, accounting for 300 deaths a year.

Prostate cancer is the second most common cancer in men, after skin cancer. One in 11 men will be afflicted with this type of cancer. This year in the United States, 132,000 new cases will be detected. Thirty-four thousand men will die of prostate cancer this year.[1]

Cancer kills more children in America than any other disease. It is projected that by the year 2010, one in every 250 persons between the ages of 15 and 45 will be a survivor of childhood cancer, representing a 300% increase. They face many risks—job discrimination, insurance discrimination, recurrence of the disease, and somber decisions about marriage and family.[2] Chances are that some of these survivors are in your congregation, perhaps in your smaller circle of concern.

The treatment of heart disease has improved dramatically. Now many people who would have died by heart attack are living longer—only to be stricken by cancer. Cancer among the over-65 crowd is on the increase.

Can't the Church Be More Helpful?

You are not alone if you think that the church is not as helpful to cancer victims as it could be. Cancer victims tell me that they know the church prays for them; some even pray in faith for miracles of healing. But beyond prayer, it seems the church does not know what to do. Not knowing what to do, many church members do nothing.

Shouldn't Christians know how to listen, to comfort, to support families of cancer victims? How many people in your church understand the fear, the helplessness, the pain cancer victims wrestle with?

There is another reason for the church to step up and minister to the personal, family, and spiritual needs of cancer victims. You might ask, "Aren't there cancer support groups in our hospitals and in community service agencies?" Yes, and they do a lot of good work. The meetings are helpful and many of the clinicians skillful. But nearly all of them have one big minus—they do not bring the Christian faith to bear on the agonies and adjustments that come to cancer victims. They do not bring faith to bear because they can't—it's against the policies and regulations of government and many private health care agencies.

Thus the cancer support groups in most community service agencies have only psychological and clinical resources to offer. Does it not then behoove the church to take a giant step forward in serving cancer victims by sharing the resources of the faith with them? No community service agency sees the meaning, purpose, and redemptive dimension of suffering that the Christian faith does.

One of the targets of this book is to bring together in "holy union" the resources of the Christian faith and the practical knowledge we have about coping with cancer. When cancer strikes a church member, the church family, as well as the biological family, struggles with the issue of suffering. The church needs to be able to assist these individuals and families in at least four areas.

1. The victims themselves or their friends sometimes question their relationship with God. Perhaps they have been drifting, taking God and their salvation for granted. Facing the threat of death earlier than expected may bring intense soul-searching. Often this is a futile search for some reason why the ill person deserves to suffer.

2. Their understanding of human suffering is challenged. When everything was going well, it was easy to sing of God's love and goodness. Now they may feel that God is punishing or torturing them, or perhaps they wonder if He really exists.

3. Their ability to cope with the grim realities of mortality is tested. Our society celebrates youth and avoids facing death. Even Christians absorb these subtle attitudes. A diagnosis of cancer creates shock to those living by such a philosophy of life.

4. Their ability to make use of medical and community support resources may be hampered by the attitude that God will heal them without any medical intervention. Sometimes this is true, but it does not always happen.

A support group made up of fellow Christian strugglers can help the cancer victim and family meet these needs.

Let's Start with the Word

Since the Bible is the story of God's dealings with people throughout time, people's lives are their stories. "Persons who have received the news of a diagnosis of cancer have a dramatic change in the plot of their story. The spiritual task ahead of them is to make sense of it."[3] The task of the church, the caring community, is to assist them with this spiritual task, since each individual story helps make up the corporate story of the church.

Jesus is the Pattern for caring. He saw each person as incomparably valuable in the eyes of God. He listened for particular needs of each person as He met him or her. He was patient with each one's growth.[4]

In the story of the healing of the deaf and mute boy, Jesus addressed the father with questions. He accepted the reply of the father when the father asked for help with his unbelief (Mark 9:14-24).

Jesus ignored the rules of the religious leaders when He healed on the Sabbath the woman "bent over" with infirmity. He touched her, and she straightened up and praised God (Luke 13:10-15).

The rich young ruler came asking what to do to inherit eternal life. Jesus engaged him in conversation and was sad that wealth meant more to the young man than following God.

At the pool of Bethesda, Jesus asked the invalid of 38 years, "Do you want to get well?" and engaged in conversation with him (John 5:1-14).

Jesus patiently taught the disciples what they would need to know after His death. He promised them that their grief would "turn to joy" because the Holy Spirit would then come (John 16:20, 13).

Paul writes that nothing can separate us from the love of God (not even cancer) because Jesus is interceding for us (Rom. 8:28-39). It is Paul who tells us to share in the burdens of others (Gal. 6:2).

If the Bible teaches us anything, it teaches us to care for each other as God in Christ cared for us. We are to meet the persons where they are and help them grow in whatever situation they find themselves when stricken by cancer.

The Bible teaches that not all who suffer have sinned. We must not assume that the person struck with cancer deserves this "judgment." Job's "comforters" did not know of the meeting between God and Satan when they accused Job of some secret sin.

The Bible teaches us that God suffers with us, that Jesus, His Son, suffered and died on the Cross. God raised Him up, but only after His purpose was served—salvation for us.

The Bible teaches us that the death of this body is inevitable. The body will return to the dust from which it came, but we have the grace of God to face that death. The promise of eternal life is ours.

The Bible teaches us that no matter how far we stray from God, we can repent and find forgiveness. It also teaches that Christians need to help each other when forgiveness is needed, rather than simply to condemn.

The Bible teaches us that it is human to have feelings, a whole range of feelings, from happiness to despair. In the Psalms we see free expression of feelings and the confidence that God hears, understands, and holds out hope.

In the chapters that follow, I want to present briefly some of the feelings of cancer victims, families, and friends or acquaintances. Then I will attempt to paint a picture of how to develop cancer support groups within the fellowship.

Part I

WHAT YOU NEED TO KNOW ABOUT PEOPLE AND CANCER

1

WHAT CANCER VICTIMS WISH YOU KNEW

They don't know how to say it politely, but there are a few things cancer victims wish you knew. You come along with your well-meant words and actions that bruise and wound. The victim may say nothing, but often he or she would like to enroll you in a remedial sensitivity class.

For ages, people have reacted to the word *cancer* as if it were a death sentence. In spite of progress made in catching the disease early and treatment bringing remission, people still react with dread and horror.

Mary had undergone surgery for cancer of the colon. Prior to the surgery she had radiation to shrink the size of the tumor, making surgery easier and giving a better chance for a "cure." One member of her church said to her, "We will sure miss your smile." Mary answered with a thank-you, but inside she thought, I'm not dead yet. The person meant well—but the words hurt Mary just the same.

Mary's story is just one example of how church people need to be sensitized and educated in how to relate to cancer victims.

"I'm not dead yet."

There is a time to let the cancer victim know how much you will miss him or her. Usually this comes at the point when everybody knows and admits that medical treatments are not working. When a person is first diagnosed, everyday activities go on as usual. The person has a hard time accepting the diagnosis. Just one day before the tests results came back, life was lurching along as usual with alarm clocks, tuna casseroles, telephone sales pitches, and obnoxious lefthand turners in traffic—all the things that make us feel jangled and normal. Then came the dreaded diagnosis. The person can't handle it—and the last thing needed is to hear some bumbling do-gooder blurt out a message of doom as if the victim had already drawn his or her last breath.

Bob lies very ill in his hospital bed, the aggressive chemotherapy treatment zapping his strength. His wife is at his bedside, as she usually is, when callers from the church come to the door of the room. They motion for her and whisper when she draws near, "How is Bob doing today?" Hesitating a little and looking back at Bob, she answers, "He is pretty weak from the chemotherapy, but he would appreciate your going over, shaking his hand, and asking him how he is doing."

Unbeknownst to the well-meaning callers, the victim is still aware of things and needs to have some control of his own situation. The ill person takes in more than you may think, and some get paranoid when the family members are called aside for a whispering conference. Give the sick person the option of responding and thus indicating how long he wishes to visit.

When questions and remarks are addressed only to family or staff in the presence of the victims, they feel that others see them as dead already. The helpless feeling already present is increased by people ignoring them. Rona, a teenager with leukemia, stated, "Sometimes I feel like the doctors aren't being honest with me when they take my parents outside of the room to talk."[1] Address questions and comments to the ill persons, and let them have control.

"Just be with me."

The ministry of presence[2] has a powerful effect, even if you can't think of anything to say. Family or friends can quietly sit in the room just to be there. Repeatedly, sick persons tell me how comforting it is to wake up and see a familiar face near at hand. Pull up those memories of childhood. Remember when you were ill and you wanted your mother right there with you? She gave you the medicine, soothed your forehead, and you drifted off to sleep. You awakened to the normal clanging noises, brother and sister fighting, and saw your mother and father in their usual places. You felt secure—you were being cared for.

The Psalmist David wrote, "Even though I walk through the valley of the shadow of death, I will fear no evil, for you are with me; your rod and your staff, they comfort me" (23:4). Just knowing God is present is comforting. As a member of the congregation, you represent God when visiting the sick person. God cares through your presence.

Several years ago I made a surprise visit to see one of my uncles in a hospital in Denver. His stepson had called to let me know that his father was dying of lung cancer, but my uncle didn't want him to let any of the rest of the family know until after he died. When I arrived, the nurses pointed out what room was his, and I sat down in the chair near his bed. When he awoke and saw me, he began to cry softly. In a whisper, due to the effects of radiation treatments, he asked, "What are you doing here? There's nothing you can do." My response was, "About the cancer, true, but I can be here for you." The tears *really* flowed then.

That weekend I sat in the chair and either read, wrote letters, wrote in my journal, or talked with him when he was awake. The nurse said how glad he was to know that my uncle had family and that I had come. My uncle never finished his six weeks of radiation. He went home with his stepson to live until he died.

"Let me express my feelings, however irrational."

Amy Harwell writes of the emotional roller coaster on which a cancer victim rides. She states that these feelings are not always based on rational facts, so that attempts to answer, even with great promises from the Bible, can feel like an affront to the ill person. It is a tall order, says Harwell, for a friend to hang in there and allow the person to ride the roller coaster to the finish. She adds that finally an adjustment to reality takes over, and the person "lives until he dies."[3]

Listening is very important. The person who is talking hears his or her own words and makes adjustments accordingly. To allow the person this opportunity is a great gift (and hard to do when we think we know the answers).

Lillie went to the doctor because she had been tired for so long. She couldn't remember how long. After tests, the verdict came back that she had lymphoma in late stages. Her friend from church came to visit her shortly after Lillie received the diagnosis.

LILLIE: I'm mad at God. I've lived a good life, I've done the best I knew to do. Why would God let this happen to me?

FRIEND *(startled at the expression of anger toward God but feeling checked by the Spirit to give an answer):* Are you asking me for an answer, or do you need to talk about feelings?

LILLIE *(starting to cry):* I need to talk. I know God is not out to zap Christians, but it doesn't seem fair that the Christian suffers while the wicked person sails through life in ease.

FRIEND: Oh, Lillie, I try to imagine myself in your spot, and I think *I* would be very upset. How would I cope?

LILLIE: Well, I've been thinking . . . the idea that comes to me is to read the Psalms. The Bible says that David was a man after God's own heart, yet bad things came David's way. The Psalms tell of David's feelings but end in praise to God. Maybe I can praise God again after talking about my feelings.

FRIEND *(with tears in her eyes):* I hope so, Lillie. I think of the 42nd psalm, where it says that "my tears have been my food day and night." It ends something like "I will yet praise him."

Most people who have been Christians a while have stored in their memory helpful Bible verses and statements of belief. Pulling together the ones appropriate for the present situation escapes them. You, as listener, serve the function of helping the victim pull out what is in his or her memory. What a great function!

Jane had been diagnosed with ovarian cancer, which had already spread to other body organs. At 35 years of age, with three little children, and a husband who aspired to climb the corporate ladder, Jane felt overwhelmed. Mrs. Dear came to visit her, representing the congregation, and after a few comments about the weather and other pleasantries, Jane started to express some of her feelings.

JANE: I feel so heavy, so depressed. I'm only 35 and have this awful disease . . . *(trailing off).*

(Although MRS. DEAR *wanted to say that* JANE *should not feel that way, she remembered what was said in the lay ministry class and silently waited for* JANE *to continue.)*

JANE: I won't be able to take care of my family, to see Jim succeed and the children grow up *(cries).*

*(*MRS. DEAR *reaches for* JANE's *hand, gets tears in her own eyes, and nods her head.)*

JANE *(regaining some composure):* I always thought that was the task for a Christian woman, like it says in Proverbs—you know the chapter that's always read on Mother's Day?

(MRS. DEAR *nods her head and looks at* JANE.)

JANE: Somehow I feel like a failure, even though I know it sounds crazy. Maybe I am paying for sins before becoming a Christian, or maybe I've had some secret sin my conscious mind won't face, or . . . *(trails off)*.

MRS. DEAR: I can't picture that, but how do you plan to sort it all out?

JANE *(reflectively):* I think I can talk to God like I am talking to you. *(Pause)* God says the Holy Spirit is within us to reveal things to us when we ask. *(Pause)* Thanks for coming and listening. I feel like I am on my way to finding peace with God.

Mrs. Dear did not say much out loud, but she said quite a lot with her mouth shut. She said that it was all right to own your feelings and to express them to God as well as to others.

The human body is basically a communication center. "Every nerve, organ, function, thought, act, tissue is a transmitter and receiver."[4] A person is whole only as another person listens, understands, and then responds. A person "cracks up" when no one listens. The power source of the communication center is love.[5] And love is sometimes best expressed by *anointed listening.*

The church means to be there for people, but without an organized way to do that, some people get forgotten. Saying hello to each other before or after church service is only a tiny part of showing love. Several guidelines for listening with the heart are summarized in figure 1.

Figure 1

LISTENING HINTS

1. Ask open-ended questions.
   How are things going for you?
   How does that feel to you?
   How would you describe your relationship with God?
   What would you like your relationship to be?

2. Use silence and/or body language as a response.

   VICTIM: I feel God is so far away if there even *is* a God.

   (You look into the victim's eyes, leaning forward to touch his or her arm, waiting expectantly.)

   VICTIM: Do you ever wonder if God really exists?

   (Still looking into the victim's eyes, you nod.)

   VICTIM: Wow—you mean I'm not weird? *(Starts to cry and laugh at the same time)*

3. Listen for themes, such as fear, abandonment, anger, guilt, hopelessness, and then facilitate exploration. Under No. 2, above, the person expressed a sense of abandonment, with fear of being weird as a secondary theme.

   VICTIM: I must have done something to bring this punishment from God.

   YOU: In reflecting on your life, has God pointed out any sins to you?

   VICTIM: No, I can't think of anything, except maybe not eating right, or sometimes I didn't want to go to church or have devotions.

   YOU: When you reflected on these things, how did you resolve them?

   VICTIM: I don't know.

   YOU: How would you like things to be?

   VICTIM *(crying):* I want to be right with God.

4. Clarify your own understanding of what you heard the person say.

You: Let me see if I understand what you have been saying. *(Then summarize the issue or issues expressed.)* You feel afraid that you are not really saved, that if you died now you would be lost—am I hearing correctly?

5. Do something with what you hear.

Victim *(crying):* I want to be right with God.

You: Let's tell God that now. May I pray with you about it?

Victim: Please.

(See figure 2 for sample prayers.)

2

FOUR MORE THINGS CANCER VICTIMS WISH YOU KNEW

Concerns galore reside in the hearts of cancer victims. I want to present four more of these concerns so that you may know at least some of the hurts felt by the cancer victim.

"It hurts when you won't touch me."

Dean had leukemia and was hospitalized for blood transfusions. A friend, Louis, came to call. Louis stopped by the nurse's station to ask if it was all right to visit his friend. The nurse nodded and then added, "If Dean is asleep, wake him up. Visitors are good therapy." So Louis went to the room. Sure enough, he had to wake Dean up, but the smile on Dean's face erased the uneasy feelings. Louis pulled up a chair at the bedside and sat down. Dean extended a hand, which Louis grasped firmly. They talked for about 10 minutes before Louis had to go.

Dean reflected afterward about an earlier visitor who had stayed in the doorway saying, "I have only a minute to visit." Dean wondered if a sign hung on his door that read, "Do Not Touch—Contagious," but now he knew that was not so. Louis had come to the bedside and even grasped his hand.

A lot of people have a fear of cancer being contagious, thinking that somehow they could "catch" it. Back in the late 1950s, one church was required to either sell the parsonage or have it fumigated. The wives of the two previous pastors had been diagnosed with and died of the same type of cancer after living in the house.

An older woman was hospitalized in the terminal stages of cancer. Her daughter-in-law came to the hospital nearly every day to visit. When she came home, her husband made her shower and change clothes out on the enclosed back porch. Only then could she enter the house and interact with him and the boys. This man feared catching cancer so much that he would not visit his own mother. After her death, he would not allow any of her possessions to be brought into his house.

One man complained, "My wife won't kiss me anymore. She thinks cancer is catching." According to the National Institutes of Health, the fear of cancer being contagious is widespread. Many people do not say this out loud, but they let their actions do the speaking. Some spouses avoid sexual contact under the guise of not wanting to hurt the victim. Many cancer victims fear that their mates are unfaithful but do not say it aloud.

Fear of contagion is destructive. It infects every area of a relationship. Even though the fear is unfounded, it is hard to help the frightened person. In the meantime, the ill person is cut off and may feel like quitting the struggle to get well. If loved ones and friends keep them at a distance, why try?

The phone rang, and Mary picked up the receiver. The caller said, "Mary, you've been on my mind. We must get together." Mary and her friend exchanged a few more bits of information about how chemotherapy was going and said good-bye. But the getting together never happened. Mary felt that others considered her to be contagious; the only contact was by phone. How could she get the hugs she needed to cope?

Touch is important for adults as well as children, but

we tend to give up tender exchanges as childish stuff. The only exception seems to be the marital relationship, and in today's society that is often mere sex rather than tender exchanges.

Research is being done concering the effect on adult health of touch during a person's infancy. Jeff Miller writes of research being done at the University of California at San Francisco.[1] For 18 years, Sandra Weiss, a nurse researcher in the School of Nursing, has been studying the effects of touch in the newborn, especially premature babies. She has concluded that touch is a powerful catalyst affecting everything from heart rate and blood pressure to self-esteem and body image. "Touch is the first language we learn when we enter the world."[2]

Touch is a "way to define self and experience the world."[3] For years we have known that infants taken care of methodically but without tender loving care do not survive. Studies demonstrate that touch improves visual perception, physiological functions, and body concept. Animal studies suggest that the type and location of touch early in life affect neural connections in the brain that are closely tied to behavior and cognitive skills.[4]

Further, the skin is the largest organ in the body, weighing 8 to 10 pounds and covering nearly 20 square feet. It regularly renews itself and houses sensory receptors that constitute touch. If our brain registered every felt touch, it would be overwhelming. The brain screens out some of these touches.[5]

The Psalmist David exclaims, "I praise you because I am fearfully and wonderfully made; your works are wonderful, I know that full well" (139:14). Research studies are bearing this out.

In looking at the life of Jesus, the tone is one of tender touch. "O Jerusalem, Jerusalem, you who kill the prophets . . . how often I have longed to gather your children together, as a hen gathers her chicks under her wings" (Matt.

23:37). Jesus even touched the man with leprosy who came to Him on his knees. "Filled with compassion, Jesus reached out his hand and touched the man" (Mark 1:41). Even though the crowds were almost "crushing" Him, Jesus knew when the hem of His garment was touched by the woman who had been bleeding for 12 years. He said, "Who touched me?" (Luke 8:45).

"Pray with me. Do you know how to help me pray?"

Prayer can be the most comforting act and the hardest act to perform when one is seriously ill. Scripture teaches that the Holy Spirit prompts us to pray and directs petitions. He also "intercedes for us with sighs too deep for words" when we "do not know how to pray as we ought" (Rom. 8:26, RSV).[6] The victims, in their anxiety over the illness, feel guilty about not praying appropriately. You are needed to remind them of this work of the Holy Spirit. You also help when you pray out loud with them. Sample prayers are given in figure 2.

Figure 2

Sample Prayers

These prayers are given as general rules. You can personalize the prayer according to the concerns presented by the person you are listening to at the moment.

Assurance of Salvation

O God, You know us better than we know ourselves. You love us with an everlasting love. *Richard* wants to make sure he is right with You. If there are some things he needs to confess now, show those to him so that he can repent and receive forgiveness. *(Pause)* If everything is all right with him, give him the assurance of the Holy Spirit. May he use Your energy to fight the cancer. Amen.

Concern for Family

God, our Creator and Guide through life, meet with us now. *Jane* is concerned about her family and how they will survive when she is gone. You know the struggles of each of them, of *John* with his high-stress job, of *Jim* still in high school trying to make sense of life, of *Lisa* just six years old and not able to understand why Mom is so ill. Put Your arms of love around each one to comfort them as they face this trial together. Grant them the freedom to say to each other what is in their hearts. We rest in Your grace. In Jesus' name we pray. Amen.

Discouragement

Lord, *June* is feeling discouraged today. The chemotherapy is making her very ill, her hair is coming out, her children are having to wear gowns and masks to visit her so that she will not catch any germs, and there are many other frustrations. I lift her up to You right now for the comfort only You can bring. May she feel the warmth of Your touch throughout her body right now. May she rest in Your arms as she did in her mother's arms as a child. We rest in Jesus' name. Amen.

Financial Concerns

God, *Bob* feels such a burden for the physical welfare of his family. The cancer treatments cost so much, and they have barely enough under normal circumstances. The insurance covers 80 percent, but the rest is still enormous. He can't go back to work and feels helpless, as if he is at fault for having cancer. Lord, You own the cattle on a thousand hills, and You invited us to come with our needs. We come now with this need and ask for Your help. May *Bob* release his feelings of guilt over not being able to work. Lord, bless this family in their many struggles, for Jesus' sake. Amen.

Robert Morris indicates that our culture considers anxiety indicative of abnormality, weakness, or maladaption. He says Christian tradition hints that anxiety is a basic ingredient of human experience and that anxiety can be an ally. "Do not be anxious about tomorrow, for tomorrow will be anxious for itself. Let the day's own trouble be sufficient for the day" (Matt. 6:34, RSV). Morris interprets this as not saying no to anxiety, just no to anxiety regarding tomorrow. It implies concern for today.[7] Deal with the *now.* Take one day at a time.

Morris relates part of a conversation between a pastor and a member of his congregation, the mother of a six-year-old with a malignant brain tumor.

MOTHER: On Tuesday they found out the tumor was growing again.

PASTOR: Oh, I am sorry to hear that.

MOTHER: Yeah . . . he's felt miserable all week. He can't walk or do much of anything. Is it all right to feel angry? I haven't felt anything for the longest time. I had to keep it all in or I'd just quit . . . I can't understand why this is happening.

PASTOR: You feel really angry.

MOTHER: I'm worried about it though.

PASTOR: I think it's OK to feel angry. It's a terrible thing he is living with.

MOTHER: Well, that's just it. Why is God letting this happen? I mean God didn't make it happen, but I guess he's letting it happen.

PASTOR: That must feel horrible.

MOTHER: Well, I've tried to think if I haven't been faithful enough. If I had more faith, maybe this wouldn't have happened. I don't know what I'm going to do when he dies. I'm afraid I'll turn away from God altogether.

PASTOR: That feels scary.

MOTHER: Yeah. Do you think it's OK to be angry?

PASTOR: I'd be angry too. It's OK to be angry with God.[8]

There are two themes in this conversation: anger toward God and anxiety over expressing that anger. Although the woman's pastor seemed to validate that it is OK to be angry with God, a verbal prayer with her might have solidified the OK. It need not be a long prayer. Taking her hand while praying makes it even better. "Lord, You know the stress that Mrs. M. has been under and the many feelings she has experienced, including anger. You also know her concern at expressing that anger to You. Right now, put Your loving arms around her and let her know You understand. Give her strength for the hard times yet ahead for her and young Timmy. Thank You. Amen."

Chances are she will cry as she feels the warmth of God's arms around her. This prayer experience will be relived when needed, perhaps in the middle of the night. You might even say to the person, "When you are alone and you feel the need for prayer, remember our prayer together. God will come."

"Ask me what I need right now."

If you say to me, "Call me if you need anything," I will probably not call. If you say, "I have some free time this afternoon—I will be over about 2 P.M. to help you with some of the housework or whatever you decide is important to you at the time," I will feel relieved and look forward to seeing you. I don't want to be a burden to anyone.

In answer to my question, "What was helpful to you after your surgery for cancer?" Wanda said, "My friend came to my house and said she was going to clean for me and that I was to lie down and rest. I did just that." But not everyone wants a friend to just take over. If you are a close friend of a cancer patient, you may be able to discern what is best. If not, ask what the sick person would like for you to do right now.

There is a variety of things you can do that will help the victim. One of those may be singing hymns with—and not to—him or her. Some comforting hymns are (1) "A Shelter in the Time of Storm," (2) "Great Is Thy Faithfulness," (3) "It Is Well with My Soul," (4) "Day by Day," (5) "Under His Wings," (6) "Rock of Ages," and (7) "How Great Thou Art." If you feel the need to have a tape playing, make sure you still sing with it. Active participation is important for the sick person to gain the optimum benefit. Take a hymnbook with you and ask the cancer patient to name some of his or her favorites.

The Psalms speak a lot about singing and making music to the Lord. Reading some of the psalms to the ill person can be very comforting. A tape of the psalms may be helpful, but only if the person has to be alone. Part of the value of hearing is that a person, a warm and caring person, is there in the room with them while reading God's Word. Do not underestimate the value of your presence.

Due to side effects of chemotherapy for leukemia, Mr. Zee had a stroke. His speech became slurred and one side of his body weakened. The speech therapist told Mr. Zee's wife to bring a book of familiar songs. They were to spend half an hour a day in singing to help his speech clear up. She brought a hymnal, since it contained the songs most familiar to them both. He would grumble, then she would tell him, "OK, if you don't want to get better, we won't sing." He would then sing with her. Of course, she had to shut the door because he didn't want anyone to hear his feeble attempts at singing. He did get better.

"Don't forget your sense of humor."

"A merry heart doeth good like a medicine" (Prov. 17:22, KJV). Modern studies are validating that laughter releases positive healing forces in the body. A short item on the bulletin board of a cancer unit indicated that a person needs 15 laughs a day to stay healthy. It concludes with the words "Go ahead and laugh; it's good for you."

Kathleen Keller Passanisi describes in her workshop several physiological and psychological benefits of laughter or humor. Laughter increases circulation and respiration, decreases blood pressure and muscle tension, causes secretion of alertness hormones, and encourages the secretion of tears with lysozymes (cleansing tears). Humor opens lines of communication, decreases anxiety and tension, keeps one alert, helps facilitate learning, stimulates creativity, helps build self-confidence, and gives one a general sense of well-being.[9]

Jesus used humor in describing the hypocrisy of those who judge others. "Why do you look at the speck of sawdust in your brother's eye and pay no attention to the plank in your own eye?" (Matt. 7:3). Picture what Jesus is saying. Use this type of humor in situations that are frustrating, when the other person is unable to change what is happening. The person who is undergoing chemotherapy and suffering side effects can use it. Hair loss can be seen as eliminating the need to comb it. The humor does not have to pertain to the disease. If you and your sick friend are used to sharing funny stories about life in general, now is no time to stop.

3

WHAT FAMILY MEMBERS OF CANCER VICTIMS WISH YOU KNEW

Too often family members are overshadowed by all the attention given the victim. It is not that you give the attention directly to the victim, but you ask a family member how the sick person is doing. You expect the family members to be unaffected, since they do not have the disease. But cancer afflicts the whole family.

"Ask how *we* are doing."

His friend asked, "How is the wife doing?" and Jim replied, "She is doing about the same." Tired, frustrated, even angry at God, Jim longed for someone to ask, "How are things going for *you*, Jim?" Not that he didn't care about Jane, but it would feel good to find someone to listen to his feelings. But Jim didn't want to ask anyone—he or she might think him weak. He and the kids seemed stuck on the sidelines.

Shirley was working at the puzzle table when I approached her and asked, "How are you doing?" She responded, "He's not too good today." I then asked, "And how are *you* doing?" She laughed a little, then answered with a sigh, "All right." It is hard for some family members to hear anything but an inquiry about the sick person.

Shirley and I then talked for about 30 minutes about her struggles.

Family members have struggles, feel burdens, get depressed, and are scared to death about the whole situation. Give them some time out, a listening heart, and relief from some of the duties at church and home.

"Please—I'm dealing with enough."

Art connected the phone to the answering machine. Most calls he did not return. When Sue finally got to talk with him, his explanation went like this: "I can't take any more of other people's sad stories. I have enough of my own." Thinking it would help, people called to share their own sad stories. He found it a burden and quit answering the phone. His wife could not walk anymore, and the pain medicine kept her in an incoherent state. His mother had just died of cancer a few months earlier after a prolonged time in a nursing home.

Art felt dumped on. Sharing of stories helps in the right place and with the proper timing. A support group provides the atmosphere to allow sharing by all those present. Calling individually on the phone to tell your tragic story feels different. It might be beneficial if attentiveness to Art came first.

The family members do not want to seem ungrateful; thus they listen patiently—at least outwardly. You want to focus on the concerns of the family member you are talking with right then.

"We have fears too."

Recalling how her uncle had died from prostate cancer with metastases to the bones, Rose pictured her husband, Ron, in that horrible state. Ron had just been told that he had cancer of the testicles. He didn't want to talk about it, acting as if everything would be just fine. Rose could not feel that way but went along with Ron's silence.

How Rose longed for someone to listen to her fears and hold her in his or her arms! Her father told her to keep a stiff upper lip, that Ron would be fine. Her mother just cried and left the room when Rose tried to talk with her. Their four-year-old son said, "Daddy's going to be OK, isn't he, Mommy?" Of course, she nodded. She did not trust herself to speak without crying. She knew Ron would not like her crying in front of their son. And she didn't want to burden a four-year-old. Whom could Rose talk to about her fears?

You could be a friend to Rose, listening to her fears. You could find out about support groups for her and even go with her to the group. Hopefully a support group meets at your church, but if not, you could start one or find one in the community.

Usually the family members have fears regarding how long their loved one has to live. Although the person is not dead yet, the diagnosis of cancer often spells death to family members. There is a positive purpose in facing the projected loss. We do not really live until we face death. This affliction of cancer in the family provides opportunity to face death. We will all face death at some point whether it comes from cancer or old age.

When asked questions like, "What have you gained from Jim's having cancer?" the whole family often answers, "We are closer to each other. Our priorities are different now." Without help in facing the fear of death, families will not be able to say this.

"Let me have my tears."

Mildred Tengbom, whose husband had cancer, stated, "Let your tears wash clean the glasses through which you look at life."[1] She related how looking at the world through her tears, when her husband was hospitalized for surgery, changed her. She was enabled to cherish loved ones more each day, to watch for God in everyday events, and to long for a deeper knowledge of Him.[2]

Psalm 126:5 says, "Those who sow in tears will reap with songs of joy." There is something about tears that yield a refreshing feeling after they stop. Tengbom quotes Augustine: "The tears . . . streamed down, and I let them flow as freely as they would, making of them a pillow for my heart. On them it rested."[3]

After years of observation, I am convinced that tears are the safety valve for emotions, all kinds of emotions. If you laugh too much, you cry. If you are suddenly frightened, you may cry. If you are overjoyed at seeing a loved one, you cry. Tears of sadness, tears of joy, tears of grief all bring release.

Sara went along with her husband, Bill, who expressed a positive outlook, even though he had colon cancer. He had chosen not to take chemotherapy, even though evidence of the cancer spreading to the liver was seen during surgery. But when Bill wasn't around, Sara called her friends to talk of her fears and to cry with them. One day Bill overheard her on the phone. After putting down the receiver, she leveled with him about her difficult times thinking of how things would be with him gone. They cried in each other's arms. This was the beginning of a deeper relationship that helped her after his death. So much energy had been wasted to fight back tears.

A little girl dying of leukemia asked a nurse for a crying doll. Puzzled, the nurse asked, "Why do you want a doll that can cry?" "Because I think Mommy and I need to cry," the little girl said. "Mommy won't cry in front of me, and I can't cry if Mommy doesn't. If we had a crying doll, all three of us could cry together. I think we'd feel better then."[4] How wise and how honest young children are!

"Forgive me when I act crazy."

"My dad always gets mad when any of us gets sick. My mother says it's because he feels so helpless."[5] Michelle is a teenager with leukemia. The display of anger by her father is not unusual in the face of helplessness. Parents feel especially helpless when their children get sick. In fact, guilt feelings often lurk beneath the anger. After all, parents are supposed to protect their children. It's as if this disease is telling others what lousy parents they are.

When the parents are Christians, they often wonder if their past sins are bringing punishment upon their children. Anger toward God often results.

"My brothers resent the attention I've gotten since I've been sick."[6] Brad, a teenager with leukemia, brings up the problem for other children in the family. Brothers and sisters get tired of being asked how the sick person is doing and no concern for them shown. Sibling rivalry is hard enough under normal circumstances. Listen to the children.

"But Jesus called the children to him and said, 'Let the little children come to me, and do not hinder them, for the kingdom of God belongs to such as these'" (Luke 18:16). Because the parents are so stressed out, it feels as though the other children are acting up just to upset them. You can help relieve the situation by befriending the children. Take them out for ice cream or a soft drink. Allow them to talk about their feelings or whatever they want to talk about. If they do not want to talk, play a game with them. They need to have someone pay attention to them at a time when the sick family member seems to be the center of attention. You can be the presence of Jesus to these children.

4

WHAT FRIENDS AND ACQUAINTANCES OF CANCER VICTIMS WANT TO KNOW

Connie hears the prayer request at church for June. The test shouted, "Cancer." She gets a sinking feeling in the pit of her stomach. She thinks to herself, I must call June. A whole school of little butterflies flutter inside. She is afraid she will say the wrong thing, and so she puts off calling her friend.

"Help us know what to say."

Two weeks had passed since June was put on the prayer chain. She had already had the mastectomy for breast cancer. June wondered why she hadn't heard from her friend Connie. Finally, June called Connie. Connie's response: "Oh, June, I didn't know what to say, and I didn't want to upset you."

June had attended a support group while in the hospital, where she learned that sometimes the person with cancer has to initiate the call to friends. She had to let people know that it is OK to talk about cancer with her. She had to let them know she wouldn't break down, that her tears are healthful and not caused by what they said.

A relationship is a two-way street. Both parties have a responsibility for keeping it going. The cancer victim does not lose all ability to think or handle awkward moments.

In fact, he or she does not lose interest in current events, whether they are negative or positive events.

"Help us understand our avoidance impulse."

It is hard for us to see you cry or look sad. When you start to talk about your situation, we tend to change the subject to something more pleasant. We don't mean to cut you off, but we learned to do that from others as we grew up. We really do want to be of help to you.

A lot of people share such feelings when a friend is diagnosed with cancer. It is hard to change patterns of a lifetime overnight. They need help to do so.

In the context of friendship, tell your friend what you long for and need from him or her to help you cope with this tragedy. When talking with your friends, stop them if they change the subject just as you bring up negative feelings. Review with each other what friendship means—honesty in the relationship. Either one of you may feel hurt when some thoughts are shared, but the air is cleared for building a more solid relationship.

I have often gone to visit a sick friend and have come away feeling I received more help than I gave. For a relationship to continue and deepen, both persons must benefit. The relationship turns sour if one person does all the giving and the other person does all the receiving. The sick person will contribute to the relationship when given the opportunity.

"Help us face the reality of death."

John became quite ill at ease as he listened to his friend, Bob. Bob described his fears that the medicine would not stop the cancer and then he would die. John could not identify all the sources of his anxiety. He knew part of the concern was that he did not want his friend to die. Then he remembered the class he had taken in college on death and dying. He knew he did not want to face his own death and that it could just as easily be he instead of

Bob with the cancer. We're both too young to die, he thought. John and Bob were 30-year-olds.

Bob noticed that John had stopped listening. He waited a minute, then asked, "John, what's bothering you?" John then shared with Bob the discovery about the cause of his anxiety. They both then talked of what it might be like to die and what it might be like for the other one to die first. They talked about how their family members might react at their loss. It was uncomfortable at times, but the results were liberating.

It is so easy to cover up our feelings about death with statements about how great heaven will be. It is also easy to avoid our feelings by claiming that God is going to heal us or the one we love whether by medicine or by miracle. Many people think, consciously or unconsciously, that considering death as a possible outcome of this cancer is tantamount to causing their own deaths. They believe that faith for healing excludes allowing for the possibility of death.

Most people who share with family and friends their feelings about death discover it frees them to really live. They have more energy to work with the medicine and with God to fight the cancer. Fighting against feelings takes much energy.

The cancer victim looks so fragile.

Most people visit the sick person while he or she is in the hospital. Often the scene includes all kinds of tubes hooked up to the person lying in the bed. Due to exhausting procedures and tests, treatments, and the meaning of the news of cancer, the person in bed does look fragile. But each of them wants to have the opportunity to visit with friends and set the limits of conversation or activity.

When treatment is finished, strength returns and activities should resume as normal. Friends tend to want to do everything for the cancer victim, which may not be good for the person. A good friend asks what would be helpful and then follows through with the answer.

Part II

WHAT YOU NEED TO KNOW ABOUT THE CHRISTIAN FAITH

5

WHAT YOU NEED TO KNOW ABOUT GOD AND SUFFERING

Joy, 31-year-old wife, mother of 4- and 6-year-old boys, member of a "house church," lay there with her eyes closed and the soft sound of Christian music in the background. She was now blind and bruised; the leukemia and chemotherapy side effects had combined to completely ravage her body. She could no longer play her guitar or go out to the "quiet room" to read or pray. Due to an extremely low blood count, she was in isolation to protect her from the germs of others. Her boys had been told in a family conference that if Mommy did not get well, it was not God's fault. She explained to them that Mommy evidently did not understand God when she thought He was going to heal her.

At age 29 Joy came to the hospital for the initial chemotherapy treatment for leukemia. Many months prior she knew something was seriously wrong because of the extreme, unexplained fatigue. As she prayed about the situation, God told her it would all work out fine. She interpreted this as a promise of healing. Joy and the medical staff would work cooperatively with God, according to Joy.

The first hospitalization extended to two months, the treatment being very aggressive. Joy talked of her faith for healing and how the fellowship of believers took care of her husband and boys. People in the church signed up for providing supper, doing the laundry, taking care of the boys, cleaning the house, and anything else that needed doing. Different ones from the fellowship visited her and prayed with her. Her faith remained deep in spite of the side effects of treatment.

Through the first to almost the last of the many hospitalizations, Joy brought her guitar and the tapes of Christian music. If the staff heard singing accompanied by a guitar, it would be Joy expressing her faith. She attended the hospital support groups and inspired others in attendance. She shared her human emotions, such as her frustrations and discomfort from being unable to care for her own family, but she also expressed her deeper "knowledge" that God was going to heal her.

During the course of the treatments, Joy talked of her estrangement with her family of origin. Her childhood had been very difficult. Someone contacted her father, who came to see her. After many years, a reconciliation with her father had begun. This was one of the positives in a negative situation.

During one of the long hospitalizations when Joy had to be in isolation for her own protection, the staff wanted to help reduce the feeling of isolation. The boys had colds and could not come to visit their mom. The equipment was gathered, and a video was made from Joy to her boys. With the help of their dad, the boys made one to send back to her.

The church fellowship continued to actively support and help the family through almost two years of this illness. The doctors finally told Joy that the chemotherapy was not putting the disease into remission and suggested discontinuing it. She and her husband agreed. She came in only when she needed blood transfusions. It was at this point that the family meetings included the boys, and everyone cried together. Faith that God was still going to heal physically remained, but the idea that He might not do so was finally faced. Joy did not want the boys to be angry with God or to blame Him. She tried to teach them that human understanding is limited. Joy died.

Based on biblical principles, how would you have handled the situation? As a victim? As a family member? As a friend? What is important when a Christian is stricken with cancer? How can we maintain our faith in a loving God when undeserved suffering is all around us? Where was God for Joy? For her family? What was God's relationship to Joy's suffering?

"Why do good people suffer?" "Why does a good Christian suffer?" We will never have a complete answer to these questions in this life, but we can consider what the Bible says about the mystery of suffering and what biblical scholars have found in their studies.

Reflecting on God and Human Suffering

A perplexing triangle exists when trying to speak justly of God when faced with awesome suffering. The three sides of the triangle are: (1) God is unsurpassingly good, (2) God is incomparably powerful, and (3) suffering and evil nonetheless exist—why?[1]

Through the centuries since the death and resurrection of Christ, Christians have grappled with the problem of suffering and evil. Consider these 12 basic pastoral consolations condensed from theologian Thomas Oden.

1. God does not directly will suffering. God works to amend what has become broken in His creation.

2. God's great gift to us is free will. It carries with it the possibility of abuse.

3. God's power can draw good out of evil. Adam's fall was a "blessed disaster" in that it was the occasion for God to bring redemption in Jesus Christ. The good is not always on an individual level but on the societal level.

4. Evil does not limit God's power. Only God could permit and welcome other freedoms.

5. Lessons of affliction come with suffering. Capacity for compassion is increased and awakening of conscience comes from suffering. Caution is required because this point can be easily distorted.

6. There are cleansing and educative elements of suffering. Chastisement meant help through cleansing (Luke 13:4-5). Suffering disciplines us, it weans us away from idolatries to trust God more, but it should not be thought of as punishment.

7. Individual suffering is socially rooted and socially redeemed. We suffer from our own and others' sins plus from things that happened long ago. We also receive benefits from the good done by people in the past.

8. Suffering may put goodness in bolder relief. There can be an increased capacity for joy. Still, suffering should not be sought in order to wring the "joy" out of it.

9. The values are intrinsic to the struggle. We grow from oppositions, tension, and struggle.

10. Proportional receptivity of the good is found. God gives His goodness according to our capacity to receive it.

11. Evil is a privation of the good. One cannot have sickness unless one had health. For example, cancer is too much of a good thing, the capacity for cellular division.

12. Is this world the best God could do? God chooses the world best for the whole.[2]

People around the world still have problems trying to fit together the fact that God is love while so much evil and suffering exist. A Japanese girl in Tokyo says, "If there is a God, why is there so much suffering in the world? Especially, why do the innocent suffer?"[3] Faith in God is often thrown away because of the depth and extent of human suffering in the world today. Alleviating human suffering assumes highest value, requiring huge amounts of money for research and for treatment.

Many Christians charge God with the hurts of life. If the only view of the Christian faith a person has is an optimistic one, wherein believers are exempt from the problems that face all humanity, such a faith may be rejected in the face of real suffering.[4]

We often call suffering a problem, but it is a mystery. A problem is an issue outside of oneself to which a solution can be discovered. A mystery is an issue in which one is personally involved and from which no objective solution can be found—only a living resolution. We cannot solve a mystery, but we can resolve to live it. No complete answer will be found.[5]

There is an answer to be found to a different question. How may we suffer triumphantly? This question has an answer. It begins at the cross of Christ. God himself suffers; He does not inflict suffering. The death of Christ is the historical expression of the agony of God. You might ask, "Why would *God* suffer?" It is because of love, and it is the nature of love to give of oneself for the sake of the loved one. This takes the Cross with utter seriousness.[6]

But why does God limit himself to certain conditions that are essential to life that may cause suffering? Some things must be counted on—the sun must rise, and the seasons change. Forces may collide and cause suffering. "But because we know that God knows [our troubles], and cares, and can do something about it, we know a quiet joy even in the midst of trouble."[7]

So what can God do? He can help us take misfortunes and either overcome them or make the most of them. God fulfills His purpose not in spite of but through suffering. This is the redemptive use of our suffering.[8]

So how does God want us to use our suffering? How can we make the most of it? We look at Rom. 8:28: "And we know that in all things God works for the good of those who love him, who have been called according to his purpose." The verse reveals that God did not make things happen but rather that He helps the sufferer to make use of what happens. The verse is also conditional. It is not "tit

51

for tat," but it makes sense that only those who place themselves in God's care are open to being helped.[9]

There are many ways to look at suffering, but some of them miss the biblical intent: suffering as obedience. The first is obedience to the fact that we are human beings and not God. The second is obedience to human limitations. The third is obedience to the discipline of humanity. We cannot expect to be exempt from suffering and live truthfully before God. It is so easy to want the suffering removed instantaneously, by the way of a miracle. Jesus, in the wilderness, refused to take shortcuts or subvert the purposes of the kingdom of God into a political power spectacle.[10]

The best approach to our anguish is to view it from Calvary. From this viewpoint we do not see a "casual connection" between God and our suffering. God is not the Author of suffering but the Sharer and Helper in suffering. Chester A. Pennington states it this way:

> If you take seriously the claim of the cross, you are confronted by a striking affirmation. God himself suffers. This is the first act to be considered when pondering our own suffering. Suffering is not just a human experience. Suffering is part of the experience of God. We can no longer speak as if God inflicts suffering upon mankind. He himself is involved in it. We can no longer think of suffering as punishment with which God cruelly disciplines his creatures. He himself suffers . . . In all their afflictions he is afflicted.
>
> Moreover God suffers deliberately . . . in order to accomplish his divine purpose. Once we see this we no longer ask why God makes us suffer. He doesn't. He himself suffers . . .
>
> We may still ask why, only this time on a much deeper level. Why does God suffer? . . .
>
> It is not that God causes . . . suffering to befall me in order that I may learn . . . or grow. But rather, in everything that happens he can help me learn . . . or grow . . . It is not that he makes it happen. Rather when it happens, he wants to help me make the most of it.[11]

It is the inalienable right of every person to profit by his or her own experience. In our culture, we try to protect others from the consequences of both their own mistakes and those of others. The purpose of suffering is that we might become a comfort to others. For example, Jesus predicted the crumpling of Peter and told him that later he would in turn strengthen the other disciples.[12]

The adage "Experience is a dear teacher" is highlighted in suffering, but learning is difficult while a person is in the middle of the traumatic experience. "However, being with others who suffer may enable the former sufferer to rethink his or her experience and make valid observations about that experience."[13] This happens regularly in support groups.

In the face of suffering we can either give up in despair or overcome. Three directions are important for overcoming, as seen in the Book of Job: to (1) accept the situation, (2) believe in oneself (Job never quit believing in his own goodness), and (3) have a complete belief in God (Job believed that God is Blesser). The question for Job was "How do I make the experience of suffering a gift?" He seemed to say, "God, You know it's not fair; You know I do not deserve what has happened to me."

Relief came for Job in the middle of a thunderstorm, when God came to him and said, "Stand up and be a man" (38:3, author's paraphrase). But why did God need to say this to Job? First, Job had been wallowing around in his suffering. He needed to stop and listen. Only then could God say, "Job, do the thing you do best." God then turned to Job's friends and said, "You men need prayer and need to sacrifice. I'm going to ask Job to pray for you" (42:8, author's paraphrase). So Job interceded with God on behalf of the others. Job knew how to talk with God. His recovery came with doing for others.[14]

I have seen many cancer victims exceed the life expectancy quoted by the medical team, and doing for others was a major part of their routine. When they were unable to do physical things, they had a prayer ministry—like Job?

One pastor wanted to encourage a lady in a "sea of troubles," so he told her the church would be praying for her. When she asked what they were praying for God to do, it startled him. Of course, he answered with the usual: healing if it was God's will and special mercy in pain. The woman replied, "Thank you, but please pray for one more request. Pray that I won't waste all of this suffering."[15]

We can enlist our suffering and make it work for us. God's answer to Paul included that suffering must become servant through the power of God. What happens *in* us helps determine what happens *through* us. Suffering reveals what is in our inner self, but God is still shaping us. "The Craftsman is our loving Father. We are the raw material. Suffering is the tool. Character is the product."[16]

Suffering reveals what a person believes deep down about the God of love and mercy. The Christian life is often presented as one of success, health and prosperity, and of delightful experiences. What an illusion! When suffering does come, faith can be lost. But God wants to transform it into a witness to His glory. Ponder this paraphrase of 2 Cor. 4:8-9: "We are often discouraged but never in despair, often knocked down but never knocked out, surrounded by enemies but never without a Friend."[17] The nameless Christians mentioned in the latter verses of the great faith chapter, Hebrews 11, were martyred.

Many have tried to make Rom. 8:28 a good-luck charm, thinking that "if you love God, you can overcome all your troubles and enjoy happiness and success and good fortune in life—complete satisfaction guaranteed."[18] Paul wrote the letter to Christians being slaughtered for their faith. At the end of the chapter, he points out that no tragedy can separate us from God's love, that we are more than conquerors.[19] This does not indicate that God works magic for Christians. But God gives grace and power to go through the trials.

What the cancer victim needs to know deep down in the soul is that God is Friend and Sharer in suffering, not a sadistic slavemaster. God does not vindictively pass out suffering. He redeems it.

How God Values You and Your Suffering

Your personal worth is stated and restated in the Bible—you are the object of God's love. He loves you unconditionally—nothing you have ever done has changed His love for you in the slightest degree. God loved you enough to send Jesus Christ to salvage you. Through Calvary, God is saying, "Look—I love you. I love you this much!"

Further, God created you in His own image. You may have fallen into sin—deep sin—but that image of God still lives in your deepest being. As John Wesley often declared, there are some remains of the image of God in the worst person.

The cancer victim needs to be reminded that, as the old Gene Cotton song affirmed, "God don't make no trash." The person struggling against cancer often also struggles with the feeling of abandonment. But God will not forsake you—and your ability to feel His presence is not the test of whether God is there or not. God is with you even if the tears of pain blind your senses to His presence.

One great contribution that the Christian faith brings to the cancer victim is the dignity of human beings. Each one of us is created in the image of God, and He who sees the sparrow fall will not forget or abandon us. You may be called coward, failure, or sinner, but you are more than that. You bear the mark of divinity, the very image of God. We are not mere animals—we are made in the image of God, built for eternity. Even death itself cannot rob the believer of eternal life. When the sinful world in which we live has done its worst, that is, wreaked physical death upon us, God redeems even that by changing death into a doorway to heaven, a passage to His very presence, the threshold of eternal joy.

Further, suffering offered to God can be made redemptive for us and for others. Our suffering joined with the suffering of Christ helps redeem this sin-cursed universe—even if we cannot always understand how. For the Christian, suffering is not wasted, futile, or empty.

Twelve Creative Choices

Being diagnosed with a rare form of lung cancer, John Packo, a pastor, decided to make creative choices based on biblical principles. These 12 choices he tells about on "Creative Choices" cards located at the back of his book *Coping with Cancer: Twelve Creative Choices.*

1. I did not choose cancer, but I choose to trust God for courage to cope with cancer (Joshua 1:9).

2. Cancer is a divine appointment to receive Christ's miracle of His life into one's heart (1 John 5:11-12).

3. Since our sovereign Lord permits cancer for His glory and our spiritual growth, I will glorify God and grow (Jeremiah 29:11).

4. Because Christ's death on the wondrous cross is the basis for divine healing, I choose His supernatural power to supplement my doctor's treatments (1 Peter 2:24).

5. I pick James's prescription administered by the elders of the local church, then leave the healing results to God (James 5:14-16a).

6. If I select the wonders of modern medicine, I must be prepared to manage the not-so-wonderful side effects (Matthew 9:12 and Colossians 4:14).

7. I practice positional thinking that produces power to live above tough circumstances (Ephesians 2:6).

8. When God withholds the miracle of instant healing, I humbly embrace His alternative of amazing grace that creates inner strength, and a joyous disposition (2 Corinthians 12:9).

9. I love God who specializes in the miracle of turn-

ing cancer into my ultimate spiritual good of Christlikeness (Romans 8:28-29*a*).

10. I dedicate my body to Christ and separate it from unhealthy eating habits, chemical abuse and over-exposure to sun (Psalm 139:14 and 1 Corinthians 3:16-17).

11. I accept death as the departure into heaven made possible by the resurrection of Jesus Christ from the dead (John 11:25-26*a*).

12. I celebrate the wonder of life by filling my heart with the joy of worshiping Jesus (Proverbs 17:22; Nehemiah 8:10*c*; and Revelation 5:13*b*).[20]

6

WHAT YOU NEED TO KNOW ABOUT THE FAITH COMMUNITY

Whatever else the church is, it is a called-out community of faith. The community's fellowship is called *koinonia*, That word was a Greek military term. A traveling troop of Greek soldiers always had a *koinonia*. At the end of a day's journey the captain would choose the site for the camp. One thing he designated was the *koinonia*, usually a place at the center or heart of the encampment. In the designated *koinonia*, all the resources (food, gear, and other supplies) were stored for the night.

At dawn the assembled soldiers received their orders for the new day. After they received their assignments, they would go to the *koinonia*, and from the resources of the whole group they would take whatever they needed to make it through the day.

The earliest Christians saw their fellowship as the *koinonia*, a source of faith, strength, comfort, and encouragement. In the whole group they found the wherewithal to face life, even when it hurled the fiercest persecution at them.

This early Christian model fuels the ministry of cancer support groups in the local church. This sort of joining hands and facing adversity together is in our Wesleyan heritage as well. John Wesley's system of societies, classes, and bands changed both the church and the world. These face-to-face groups rediscovered the power of the New Testament model. Nothing draws people together like shared adversity. Wesley called his small-group members "companions, on the walk to the New Jerusalem." He added that if you do not find such companions, you must "make them," for no one can "make this journey alone."

If that is true for ordinary Christians, it is doubly true for those battling cancer—they cannot make this journey alone.

Faith, Feelings, and Love Within the Church

The Church, as revealed in the New Testament, was part of a saved and saving community with a Savior. As an organized community, it was a priesthood of laity; all men and women were priests unto God (Rev. 1:6; 5:10; 1 Pet. 2:9). When the problem of the distribution of food to the Greek widows came up, the body of believers met and picked seven men to distribute the food. It was a democratic process. There was no particular structure in the first 100 years; the organization changed structure to meet apparent needs.[1]

Among many hindrances to faith are confused feelings. If feelings are confused, then faith is confused. Mind, will, and feelings are inseparably bound together. If the capacity to love and to understand are upset, the capacity for faith is shaken also.[2]

Feelings are shaped before faith is formed; therefore, it may be difficult to accept forgiveness or difficult to love. One may be afraid of other people and experience loneliness, alienation, and estrangement. It is important to bring feeling into a healthy working relationship.[3]

One cannot simply psychologize faith nor intellectualize feelings. Persons must *feel* forgiven as well as *think* themselves forgiven. In Christian experience we try to understand feelings in the light of faith to live as children of God.[4]

We need to affirm the love of God regardless of feelings. The love of God is grounded in His faithfulness, while feelings are not dependable. Affirming is equal to accepting. We accept what God does for us and return thanks and appreciation. Rom. 8:26 tells us that the Spirit helps us in our weakness "with groanings which cannot be uttered" (KJV). We ask God to help our self-understanding so that we are better able to understand others.[5]

"The church is intended to be a community of love: a community of men and women and youth who are really concerned for one another, are sensitive to one another, and able to minister to one another in the ways of love."[6] This concern would include sharing each other's joy, adversity, and compassionate service to the world.[7]

Prayer within the fellowship is important, but do we know how to pray? What is involved in prayer when a friend is sick? When you pray for a friend, think of his circumstances, such as the pain and fear of cancer, fear of surgery, how to pay the bills, how the family will fare, and the fears of the spouse. This kind of prayer is intense but is important in finding answers. The power does not lie in the prayer but in God. Self-giving is involved. Jesus prayed, "Thy will be done" (Matt. 26:42, KJV), as He faced the Cross.[8]

Sharing in one another's burdens demands serving, even as Christ came not to be served but to serve.[9] There is a high price to love. No one is too good to need help or to give it. We carry all of our own load that we can, but no more. Grace is the great leveler that knocks down pride (Gal. 6:3). We will be concerned enough to offer help and humble enough to ask for help.[10]

Suffering can cut us off from the "land of the living" so that a fellowship of suffering is needed. Suffering was set within the nourishing fellowship with Christ and fellow believers in the household of faith in the New Testament. The "household of faith" is a burden-sharing group.[11]

Sharing is more than the division of property. It is the communicating of experiences of the older to the younger, participation of the unskilled with the more skilled, and the consideration of one's achievements as those of community. We make room for one another in our hearts.[12]

Based on the story of Lazarus, people in the fellowship need to unbind each other. Suggestions for doing this are as follows: (1) Involve ourselves with each other as recorded in the Book of Acts. (2) Encourage, guide, and confront each other. It is important to listen and understand the hurts and struggles before offering counsel to others. (3) Emphasize responsibility for the present and future rather than blame for the past. Blame is like a plank of wood in our eyes, blinding us to the solution to our problems. (4) Emphasize commitment. (5) Teach and exhibit unconditional love, in the action of the will. Tragically, many of the worst wounds are inflicted by Christians and not the enemy. The church should be the hospital for the wounded.[13]

A Summary of the Gospel

In this little book we cannot treat every important Christian doctrine. It is assumed that anyone who would establish a support group for cancer victims would understand the following basic tenets of the Christian faith.

God is good, and His creation, including humanity, was good. Through human sin, evil entered the world and marred the good creation, including disruption of humanity's relationship with God and the fragmentation of the image of God in humanity.

God sent His Son to redeem humanity, to restore the relationship with God, to atone for sin, and to restore the image of God within the human heart. God has a perfect remedy for sin both as an act and a state.

Persons receive salvation by grace through faith as they confess and repent of their sin. God's saving and sanctifying grace always comes by grace through faith by the agency of the Holy Spirit.

To all those who put their trust in Christ, God gives the gift of eternal life, often expressed as "the Christian hope."

Faith Affirmations

Here are eight affirmations of faith that I believe provide a foundation for cancer support groups in the church.

1. Since God is all-powerful, good, loving, all-knowing, and spirit, we can trust even when we cannot understand the *what* and the *why* of our circumstances. After Calvary, God has a right to be trusted.

2. Since we are free, responsible, and created in the image of God, we can share in the creation of the future. The way we face our tomorrows actually helps *shape* our tomorrows. Some events may not be of our own making. The free choice of others, for good or evil, affects us. Our freedom is limited, but we can choose how we react to the problems and possibilities of life.

3. Since disease and evil were never God's intentional will, and since we share in the creation of the future, it is incumbent upon Christians to join hands with God in the healing of the victims of diseases (even cancer) and other tragedies.

4. Since God is love, He shares in our suffering as revealed in sending His Son, Jesus Christ, to suffer and die for us. When we suffer, God suffers with us.

5. Since sickness itself is not sin, the victim can take comfort in God's love and salvation. If the victim did, in some way such as an unhealthful lifestyle, contribute to the illness, forgiveness is offered with repentance. Salvation is found in a right relationship with God.

6. Since God created human beings for fellowship

with each other as well as with their Creator, the forming of support groups within the fellowship of believers is a natural method of assisting people in crisis.

7. Since the Holy Scriptures were given to us through the wise providence of God, they are valuable in the ministry to those who suffer.

8. Since the Holy Scriptures and experience reveal that lessons are learned through suffering, mysterious though it is, suffering is redemptive. For the Christian, suffering is not wasted.

Part III

WHAT YOU NEED TO KNOW TO START A SUPPORT GROUP FOR CANCER VICTIMS IN YOUR CHURCH

7

HOW TO GET STARTED

Getting started is never easy. The idea sounds exciting but when it comes to initiating the idea in your own fellowship, you get cold feet and procrastinate. Often this is because you do not have enough directions. If you attended a support group, it probably seemed easy enough. Then you faced the details of organizing and conducting a group. Help!

Before getting a group of people together to share their experiences, it will be helpful to learn something about groups and their purposes.

What Is a Support Group?

A support group is not a course of study with a prescribed curriculum. The curriculum comes from the needs of the persons who make up the group. Although broad areas of commonality are present, each person responds in different ways to the crisis of cancer in the family. The main ingredients of the curriculum then are compassionate listening, expressing care and Christian love, sharing spiritual experiences, and reserving judgments for God.

Resources need to be considered, including people, Scriptures, Christian faith, prayer, books, pamphlets, videos, and audiotapes that relate to coping with life-threatening illnesses. Keeping in mind that the list is not exhaustive, consider some of the resources given here.

A. People

People who have been through the trauma, learned from the experiences, and would like to assist fellow strugglers will be great resources. Nothing bonds people like shared adversity. Encourage people to tell their stories. Teach them to pray for each other each day, and how to pray together in the group.

Let the people help you set the goals and objectives, for the series of support groups. Though you will have goals and objectives, you won't set lesson plans like a Sunday School teacher. Remember: the needs represented in the group are the curriculum. When I conducted a church support group, I used a presession survey to help me as a leader know some of the concerns of the participants (figure 3). This was very profitable to me and to those who filled it out.

Figure 3

Cancer Support Group
Presession Survey

What do you hope to learn or discover from this cancer support group?

Are you or a member of your family now suffering from cancer?

Does a close friend or associate of yours have cancer?

Have any of your friends or a family member died from cancer?

What type of cancer has each of the above persons had? How long?

How has coping with the disease affected the quality of relationships in your home?

How successfully have you dealt with your feelings that have arisen from this encounter with cancer?

In what ways has that encounter with cancer affected your faith, your belief in God, your devotional life, and so on?

At what points in coping with cancer in your life, family, or circle of friends have you felt most helpless? most frustrated? angry? frightened?

Have you experienced feelings and thoughts about your encounter with cancer that you have never dared to express? (circle)

YES   NO

What else would you wish to share about your experience with cancer?

B. Prayer

You might think prayer is obvious and natural. But in the first group, I experimented in the beginning by having one person close the session with prayer and then moved to having a circle of prayer. In that circle, each person prayed for the person to his or her right (plus any concerns he or she had). There had been enough sharing already to make the prayers on target for specific needs. The evaluation in the last session indicated that prayer for each other ranked high and was very much treasured.

C. Scripture

Many passages in the Bible are helpful. A few will be listed here. Some Scripture has been quoted in earlier chapters of this book. You will think of many ways to use these scriptures. You may want one session to include direct Bible study, or you may want to put key verses on the walls or on a bulletin board. You may want to have a handout with the verses on it and space for each person to make his or her own notes.

The Book of Job, especially chapters 1, 16, and 21
The Psalms, especially 18, 23, 27, 37, 42, 90, 98, 139
Eccles. 3:1-15

Matt. 6:25-34; 22:34-40; 23:37; 25:31-40; 26:36-46
Luke 8:43-48; 18:15-17
1 Cor. 12:12-27; 13:1-13
2 Cor. 1:3-7; 4:7-9
Gal. 6:1-10 (especially v. 2)
Heb. 2:9-18; 4:16; 10:19-25
James 1:2-5; 5:7-11, 13-20

D. Literature and Other Resources

You will not be giving homework, but if the group members are reading the same good sources, it will enrich the group session. The experiences shared in the books help expand the size of the group by proxy.

You might want to see if the church library has or will provide some of these books. That way, even those who cannot come to the support group can read the books and benefit.

Having a display table for the reading material at each meeting will make it easier for members of the group to take material and return it.

Books

Bombeck, Erma. *I Want to Grow Hair, I Want to Grow Up, I Want to Go to Boise.* New York: Harper and Row, 1989.

This book is great for balancing the serious and humorous. The young people who provided the data for the author reveal the strength of youth in facing adversity with humor. It will help bring a much needed perspective on the disease of cancer.

Carlson, Dwight, and Wood, Susan Carlson. *When Life Isn't Fair.* Eugene, Oreg.: Harvest House Publishers, 1989.

This book tells the story of Susan's battle with leukemia and chemotherapy. Her father shares the perspective of family concerns and beliefs that help us go through this and other tragedies.

Davis, Ron. *Gold in the Making.* Nashville: Thomas Nelson Publishers, 1983.

This book discusses our reactions to suffering and other tragedies and how we can turn them into spiritual lessons to help us grow in grace. Many illustrations in the book deal with situations involving cancer.

Harwell, Amy, with Kristine Tomasik. *When Your Friend Gets Cancer.* Wheaton, Ill.: Harold Shaw Publishers, 1987.

Amy had cancer and from that perspective shares how friends helped her. Very practical.

Nouwen, Henri. *The Wounded Healer.* Garden City, N.Y.: Doubleday and Co., 1972.

This book is good for leaders in that it describes how those who have been through brokenness are better able to help others in the healing process.

Osgood, Judy, ed. *Meditations for the Terminally Ill and Their Families.* Sunriver, Oreg.: Gilgal Publications, 1989.

This book contains short devotionals that can be used on a daily basis or read all at once. Different aspects of coping with cancer are covered in the various devotions.

Packo, John E. *Coping with Cancer.* Camp Hill, Pa.: Christian Publications, 1991.

This book relates the struggles of John, a minister, when diagnosed and treated for a rare form of lung cancer. He shares the beliefs and strategies that brought him through the experience.

Wiersbe, Warren W. *Why Us? When Bad Things Happen to God's People.* Old Tappan, N.J.: Fleming H. Revell Co., 1984.

This books deals with the problem of suffering and the beliefs that can help us cope.

Articles or Booklets

These articles or booklets provide a brief treatment of some aspect of coping for victim and/or family. They are easy to read through at one sitting, and one feels ministered to right away.

Fischer, Kathleen. "When Grief Won't Go Away." *Care Notes.* St. Meinrad, Ind.: Abbey Press, 1990.

Kelly, Melissa. "When You First Learn It's Cancer." *Care Notes.* St. Meinrad, Ind.: Abbey Press, 1991.

Siegel, Bernie. "Love Is a Medical Miracle." *Redbook,* December 1986, 110-11, 181-84.

Taking Time: Support for People with Cancer and the People Who Care About Them from American Cancer Society.

Tengbom, Mildred. "Letting Tears Bring Healing and Renewal." *Care Notes.* St. Meinrad, Ind.: Abbey Press, 1990. Published several times a year in booklet form.

"What It Is That I Have, Don't Want, Didn't Ask For, Can't Give Back, and How I Feel About It." Columbus, Ohio: Ohio State University Comprehensive Cancer Center, Leukemia Society of America. Available from American Cancer Society (feelings of young people with leukemia).

Wintz, Jack. "Making Sense out of Suffering." *Care Notes,* St. Meinrad, Ind.: Abbey Press, 1991.

Videotape

Through the Eye of a Needle, featuring Shelly Chapin, available through Dallas Christian Video, Richardson, Tex.

This videotape is the testimony of Shelly Chapin regarding her three-year struggle with a rare form of lung cancer. She lives with pain and has coped with many surgeries for recurrences. She shares songs she composed at various points in her struggles. The story is divided into three sections of about 50 minutes each and includes discussion of the stages of grief, dealing with your doctor, and perspectives on several passages of the Bible.

A friend of mine, whose sister had died of cancer several years earlier, viewed this videotape with the rest of her congregation. She related that it was as if floodlights came on as she sensed what her sister had gone through as well as what the rest of the family had gone through. She was relieved to learn some of the dynamics that had occurred among family and friends. There are a lot of people like my friend waiting for illumination in other congregations. After discovering the information, the people can better share the burdens of fellow struggling Christians.

Don't overlook the book you are now reading as a resource. This book might be an ideal resource for a new group. Each chapter could be read and discussed informally. See the next chapter for further suggestions.

Planning

Although support for cancer victims and their families includes more than having cancer support groups, the focus of this chapter is how to organize and conduct a cancer support group.

Each congregation is different, so that no one formula fits all. The need for a cancer support group depends upon the number of affected families in the congregation—or you can start a group for the community at large as well as for church members. It could be an outreach ministry. Another possibility is going together with several other churches to form support groups. Cancer statistics from the American Cancer Society indicate that three out of four families will be afflicted with cancer at some point. In considering cancer support groups, follow these steps:

A. Pastor and Church Board Approval

The pastor and board need to consider the value of

having a group as discussed in this book. Questions about who can come, at what dates, the time frame involved, funding, and leadership accountability need to be answered. When these questions have been answered, the board needs to give final approval. But don't limit the presentation to just these policy matters—emphasize the ministry potential!

B. Organization

Organization involves several tasks. The first task is selecting leaders so that they can plan dates, time, place, and other details.

1. Core of Leaders

The choice of leaders is important before going further with organizing a group. Ideally, the leaders will be persons who have themselves battled cancer in their family and want to serve others. The reason for the leaders to be from among those who have experienced such a crisis is found in Henry Nouwen's concept of the wounded healer: "Service will not be perceived as authentic unless it comes from a heart wounded by the suffering about which [the person] speaks."[1] The person who leads or even participates in the group makes his or her own wounds available as a source of healing for others.

I found from my experiences with groups that it is best to have two leaders. While one is concentrating on listening to a participant, the other leader can be observing for clues as to the needs of other members of the group. The two leaders work together to ensure that all members have opportunity to share.

In a previous group I led, only women participated. This makes me believe that a group needs to have both a male and a female leader. The men in the congregation may think support groups are for women only. Our society has reinforced the myth that men cannot cry or let others know of their needs. Actually sharing in a support group is an indication that the person has enough strength to find help in times of crisis. What others think of him or her is not the important criteria.

Although there is some value in having seperate groups for men and women, at some point the two need to share with each other the different ways of reacting and responding to the crisis of cancer.

Qualities of a good support group leader include: (1) being a grounded Christian, (2) knowing something of the Bible, (3) being able to listen, (4) being open and accepting, (5) being nonjudgmental, (6) being comfortable with dialogue (not lecture), and (7) generally caring for people. This list may sound intimidating, but a leader need not be perfect to fulfill these qualifications. I sometimes slip into lecture. When I realize what I have done, I apologize to the group and concentrate on listening.

After identifying a core of people who would qualify as leaders, select two who are willing to prepare for and conduct a group. Allow them to set dates, time, place, publicity, and schedule.

Plan a system of undershepherding whereby "pastoral" assignments within the group can be carried out. This is especially needful if your group has more than six or eight members. Assign each undershepherd or "pastor" three or four persons. The undershepherd should work at developing good relationships with the persons to whom he or she is assigned. One contact between meetings should be the minimum assignment.

2. Spiritual Preparation

Spiritual preparation of the leaders is very important both for the leaders and for the helpfulness of the group. Most persons who volunteer for leadership of a group feel inadequate. They are caring Christians who wish to give in the same measure as they have received from God. They may feel a person has to be a "supersaint" in order to be a leader. We would have a leaderless church if being a super-saint were required. The leader of a support group provides help from a fellow struggler.

As a leader, prayerfully read the scriptural resources listed earlier in this chapter. Pray for God's presence with you at every step of setting up dates, time, place, session schedules, refreshments, or whatever else might be planned.

Pray for each family in the congregation whom you know has experienced cancer or is experiencing cancer now. Pray that God will lead them to join the group if at all possible. We need each other to both give and receive spiritual help to grow through a crisis.

3. General Preparation

Go over all the resources listed in this chapter. You may want to divide some of the literature resources between the two of you to make the load manageable. You may know of other helpful materials. The ones listed in this chapter are certainly not exhaustive.

Read all of this book so that you are familiar with some of the common feelings expressed by victims, family members, or friends. When some people dare to share concerns, they really want to know if they are alone or if others feel the same. From reading this book or other testimonies, you can affirm that others have had similar feelings. Consider carefully the chapter dealing with the foundations of the Christian faith. After all, the resources of the faith is what makes a church group unique and special.

Meet together as coleaders to work out your styles of leadership. You want to come to an understanding of how you can interrupt each other if you sense someone else needs the opportunity to share. When this subject is discussed ahead of time, hurt feelings can be avoided. Plan to meet together between sessions to ask each other for feedback as to how the session felt so that midcourse corrections can be made.

In one of your meetings together, plan a schedule for the support group sessions. When I plan for a group, I try to think of goals or objectives I would like met by the end of the meeting series. I usually plan for eight sessions. These overall objectives are kept in mind for the whole time and gone over between sessions to see if adjustments need to be made. I keep in mind that the needs of the members present are more important than any preset agenda.

Figure 4 lists my overall objectives for a support group. In addition, I break those down into two or three objectives for any one session. For example, Session One had two objectives and a plan.

The participants will

1. understand and experience some of the benefits of sharing in a group of people who share both the Christian faith and the disease of cancer;
2. know that many resources exist in print that can help them between and after the sessions.

Plan:

15 minutes—Broad introduction to support groups
　　　　　　Presession survey
10 minutes—Videotape of a cancer support group
　　　　　　(brings out the benefit of "hope")
10 minutes—Refreshments
55 minutes—Sharing of own stories

Figure 4

Overall Objectives for Support Group

The participants will

1. identify some of the biblical passages that relate to suffering;
2. appreciate how some of the biblical passages help persons cope with the suffering being experienced;
3. experience the benefits of sharing feelings and concerns with others in their faith community;
4. feel more comfortable in the process of sharing feel-

ings and concerns in the group;
5. accept their own feelings and feelings of others in the experience of suffering;
6. recognize and accept the stages of grief as they apply to illness as well as death;
7. identify several resources for the cancer victim and family to find help in dealing with various aspects of the disease;
8. continue appropriating the resources of the Christian faith after the support group has concluded;
9. share with others outside of the group the value received by participating in the support group;
10. support each other between sessions, and after the formal group is finished, by prayer and sharing.

4. Publicizing the Group

The support group meetings need to be promoted during regularly scheduled announcement times, preferably three times before the group is scheduled to start.

Written promotion can be done by an announcement in the midweek newsletter and one in the Sunday bulletin. An insert in the Sunday bulletin would allow for a response on a tear-off portion. Phone numbers of the leaders should be given so that people can call for further information.

Even though you have publicized in several ways, some may respond only by personal invitation. You may have some members who are willing to call people who you know could benefit. The personal follow-up to written promotions adds to the feeling of being cared for by fellow strugglers. Some think they do not need the group and are coping well. This may be so, but they may be able to help others in the group. When they do so, they also gain from the experience.

If your group goes on for several months, or if you have several groups going at once, you may discover that a monthly newsletter would be worthwhile. Good publicity may help you get the funding you will need for books, audiotapes, videotapes, excursions, and so on.

5. Conducting the Group

Some ideas about conducting the group have already been noted, for example, making sure everyone has the opportunity to share. This bears repeating.

Keep in mind the needs of those who are present. If new ones join the group, give a brief overview of where the group has been so that they can feel included. This will also serve as a healthy review for the others, putting previous sharing into perspective.

Respect everyone's views, even though you may not agree with the conclusions. If you tersely correct them, they will not say what their real feelings are again, or they may quit the group. If their conclusions seem different, the exposure to those of others during the course of the sessions will more than likely alter them. Sometimes we are tempted to do the work of the Holy Spirit instead of waiting.

If you sense you have cut someone off during a session, speak with him or her afterward. Ask the individual for feedback and tell him or her you do not want to cut anyone off. Apologize. We all inadvertently say things that we do not mean. It means a lot to the other person to hear that acknowledged.

When listening to members of the group, try to restate what you hear them saying, including tone of voice and body language. It will help them clarify their own feelings.

Prayer during the sessions is very important. In one group I conducted, the group evaluated the prayer time in which they held hands and prayed for each other as probably the most valuable aspect of the group. This prayer time was introduced after several sessions when they had heard each others' needs.

6. Closing the Group Sessions

You may want to have a time for evaluation of the group, perhaps in writing and/or verbally in the session.

Some do not like to write, but having some questions on paper promotes some thoughts that are shared verbally with the group.

During the last two sessions, you might bring up the need for missionaries to help form groups as needed in the future. Chances are that at least several will want to help others in this same way. You could plan for a "sending service" during the last 10 minutes of the final session. It is in this way that the biblical command to bear one another's burdens is fulfilled.

8

HOW TO USE THIS BOOK AS A GUIDE FOR A SUPPORT GROUP IN YOUR CHURCH

A support group session is meant to be flexible, based on the concerns of the members present. Yet the leaders need to have some general objectives in mind lest chaos takes over. I will share some possible suggestions (not curriculum) for using this book in an 8- to 10-session support group. You need to keep in mind some general principles as well as plans for each individual session.

General Principles

1. When a group of persons have read the same material ahead, discussion is more meaningful.

2. A danger exists of sticking only to the content of any assigned reading. People need reminding that what they read is meant to trigger concerns of their own.

3. Plans need to be flexible. If it becomes apparent that members have needs in a different direction than planned, be prepared to switch the focus for the rest of the session.

4. Prayer for others has the greatest value when it is specific to the needs.

5. God wants to love others through you. Relax and let that happen!

Session by Session

Before designing each session, think about what you want to happen overall during the course of the group sessions. You could consider those objectives listed in figure 4 of this book, or create your own, specific to the needs of people in your congregation.

Session 1

Think about what you want to happen in this session. Put it down in the form of objectives, perhaps by completing the sentences below.

"What I want my group members to *feel* during the session is _____."

"What I want my group members to *understand* during the session is _____."

"What I want my group members to *do* during the session is _____."

Plan a presession survey, either the one described in figure 3 of this book or one of your own design. The survey helps both you and the group member clarify some of the concerns.

Be prepared to give a brief overview of support groups and a few ground rules. One such rule would be that no one person dominate the entire session. Each person can help by observing how another in the group is reacting to what is happening.

Think of some starter questions for discussion, but be prepared to forget them if discussion proceeds spontaneously.

Protect a period of time during the session for free sharing of whatever is on people's hearts. This is important.

Perhaps you have a Bible reading you want to share because it fits the needs of a member of the group. You could encourage members to share some of their own in future sessions. A number of Bible passages were listed in chapter 7 of this book.

Plan for a time of prayer at some point during the session, and plan it with this in mind: Prayer often brings openness to further sharing. Holding hands in a circle and praying for the person to the right of you until all are prayed for is a great help. Consider the needs of your group members.

Perhaps you can ask each member to read the introduction and chapter 1 for the next session.

As leaders, plan a meeting for debriefing, either after the session or sometime before the next session. Leaders may do this by journaling or verbalizing.

Sessions 2 through 7

Plan objectives as you did for session 1, considering what you want to happen in the realms of understanding, doing, and feeling. Some objectives will be applicable for many of the sessions.

Plan a time for feedback on readings and insights since the last session. This is not the same as the time for sharing whatever is on members' hearts.

Refreshments may be planned for a break time. Members tend to form subgroups and continue discussing feelings that came up in the group prior to the break. This is good, for it promotes further sharing. Perhaps members will want to sign up for times to bring refreshments. Keep in mind that those with cancer may have foods that disagree with treatment.

Remember to plan for a time of prayer, with some time left in the session for response.

If it helps with sharing, assign readings from chapters 3 through 6 of this book. According to your objectives, assign portions of these chapters for different sessions.

Session(s) 8 (9 or 10)

Closing sessions need some variation in objectives, so think of what you want for the members after the sessions have ended, and design the closing sessions with that in mind.

You may want to assign chapter 7 to be read before the closing session so that the members can think of sharing with others in the same measure as they have received. You may want to have a "sending service" during the last portion of the session.

Allow time for reflection on the whole experience, whether both written and verbal or just verbal. I have found that a postsession survey on paper starts the thinking that makes the verbal evaluation better.

Again, plan for prayer time. This might be good after the verbal evaluation and before a time for ending the sessions.

People need a time for good-bye to each other. It usually includes hugs all around. You might think that it is not very important because people will see each other in church, but it will not be on the same level.

As leaders, plan a debriefing session in which you can look at your overall objectives and how they were met. You will want to consider what worked and what did not. Consider the question of what to change for another group. In other words, plan a future group now while the experience is fresh for all of you.

EPILOGUE

Dee knew something was wrong—seriously wrong. She went to the doctor just as the literature said you should do. After tests were finished, the news came back that she had cancer. The doctors said the best course of action included radiation first and then surgery. She felt she could handle that. But after the surgery, she woke up with a temporary colostomy, which became very trying for her. The clincher was that now she received news of the need for chemotherapy. Why? Because the doctors had not done a certain blood test prior to the other treatments so that comparison tests could be done. Dee told the doctors about her anger and figured she had coped well.

Dee was asked to join a support group. Her response was "If I can be of help to someone else, OK." She came. Much to her surprise, after the first session she said to herself, "Dee, *you're* the one who needs the group! What do you mean you came only to help someone else?" Dee shared this insight with the others during the second session of the support group. It did indeed help the others, as well as Dee.

Who will make sure there is a group for the many other people like Dee in our congregations?

NOTES

Introduction
    1. *Cancer Facts and Figures—1992* (Atlanta: American Cancer Society, 1992).
    2. Carol Kotsubo, "Seasons of Oncology Nursing" (Workshop sponsored by Queens Medical Center Cancer Institute, Honolulu; and American Cancer Society of Hawaii, January 22-24, 1992, in Honolulu).
    3. Mark Jensen, "Some Implications of Narrative Theology for Ministry to Cancer Patients," *Journal of Pastoral Care* 38 (September 1984): 224.
    4. Thomas C. Oden, *Pastoral Theology: Essentials of Ministry* (San Francisco: Harper and Row, Publishers, 1983), 193.

Chapter 1
    1. "What It Is That I Have, Don't Want, Didn't Ask For, Can't Give Back, and How I Feel About It" (Columbus, Ohio: Ohio State University Comprehensive Cancer Center, Leukemia Society of America), 4.
    2. J. Grant Swank, Jr., "The Ministry of Being There," *Preacher's Magazine* 68 (March, April, May 1992): 14.
    3. Amy Harwell with Kristine Tomasik, *When Your Friend Gets Cancer* (Wheaton, Ill.: Harold Shaw Publishers, 1987), 31-32.
    4. Mildred Bangs Wynkoop, *A Theology of Love* (Kansas City: Beacon Hill Press of Kansas City, 1972), 141.
    5. Ibid.

Chapter 2
    1. Jeff Miller, "The First Language," *UCSF Magazine*, February 1992, 31-35.
    2. Ibid., 32.
    3. Ibid., 31.
    4. Ibid., 33.
    5. Ibid., 35.
    6. W. T. Purkiser, Richard S. Taylor, and Willard H. Taylor, *God, Man, and Salvation: A Biblical Theology* (Kansas City: Beacon Hill Press of Kansas City, 1977), 519.
    7. Robert Morris, "Caring for the Family Facing Cancer," *Christian Ministry* 14 (March 1983): 14. Copyright 1983 Christian Century Foundation.
    8. Ibid., 15. Reprinted by permission.
    9. Kathleen Keller Passanisi, lecture given as part of the Value of Life symposium, Research Medical Center, Kansas City, May 6, 1993.

Chapter 3
    1. Mildred Tengbom, "Letting Tears Bring Healing and Renewal." From *Care Notes*, copyright 1990, Abbey Press, St. Meinrad Archabbey, St. Meinrad, IN 45577. Reprinted with permission.
    2. Ibid.
    3. Ibid.
    4. Ibid.
    5. "What It Is That I Have, . . . and How I Feel About It," 8.
    6. Ibid., 7.

Chapter 5
1. Oden, *Pastoral Theology*, 223.
2. Twelve pastoral consolations from pp. 226-40 from *Pastoral Theology: Essentials of Ministry*, by Thomas C. Oden. Copyright © 1983 by Thomas C. Oden. Reprinted by permission of HarperCollins Publishers, Inc.
3. Chester A. Pennington, *Even So . . . Believe* (Nashville: Abingdon Press, 1966), 96-97.
4. Ibid., 98-99.
5. Ibid., 102.
6. Ibid., 103-5.
7. Ibid., 107-8.
8. Ibid., 108.
9. Ibid., 109-10.
10. Wayne E. Oates, *The Revelation of God in Human Suffering* (Philadelphia: Westminster Press, 1959), 35-36.
11. Pennington, *Even So . . . Believe*, 103-9. Used with permission.
12. Ibid., 37.
13. S. Denton Bassett, "Suffering S.O.S.: Toward a Theology of Suffering," *Care Giver Journal* 8 (3): 98-99, n.d.
14. Ibid., 29.
15. Warren W. Wiersbe, *Why Us? When Bad Things Happen to God's People* (Old Tappan, N.J.: Fleming H. Revell Co., 1984), 92.
16. Ibid., 105-7.
17. Ron L. Davis, *Gold in the Making* (Nashville: Thomas Nelson Publishers, 1983), 26-28.
18. Ibid., 63-64.
19. Ibid., 68-69.
20. Taken from *Coping with Cancer: Twelve Creative Choices*, by John Packo. Copyright 1991 by Christian Publications, Inc. (Camp Hill, Pa.). Used with permission.

Chapter 6
1. Purkiser, *God, Man, and Salvation*, 600-601.
2. Pennington, *Even So . . . Believe*, 62.
3. Ibid., 63-65.
4. Ibid., 66-68.
5. Ibid., 68-74.
6. Ibid., 92.
7. Ibid., 95.
8. Alan Walker, *How Jesus Helped People* (New York: Abingdon Press, 1964), 112-13.
9. David Allan Hubbard, *Galatians: Gospel of Freedom* (Waco, Tex.: Word Books, 1977), 103.
10. Ibid., 104.
11. Oates, *Revelation of God*, 35-36.
12. Ibid., 44-46.
13. Davis, *Gold in the Making*, 80-88.

Chapter 7
1. Henri Nouwen, *The Wounded Healer* (Garden City, N.Y.: Doubleday and Co., 1972), xiv.

BIBLIOGRAPHY

Bassett, S. Denton. "Suffering S.O.S.: Toward a Theology of Suffering." *Care Giver Journal* 8 (3): 22-29, n.d.

Cancer Facts and Figures—1992. Atlanta: American Cancer Society, 1992.

Davis, Ron Lee. *Gold in the Making.* Nashville: Thomas Nelson Publishers, 1983.

Harwell, Amy, with Kristine Tomasik. *When Your Friend Gets Cancer.* Wheaton, Ill.: Harold Shaw Publishers, 1987.

Hubbard, David Allan. *Galatians: Gospel of Freedom.* Waco, Tex.: Word Books, 1977.

Jensen, Mark. "Some Implications of Narrative Theology for Ministry to Cancer Patients," *Journal of Pastoral Care* 38 (September 1984), 216-25.

Kotsubo, Carol. "Seasons of Oncology Nursing," workshop by Queens Medical Center Cancer Institute, Honolulu; and American Cancer Society of Hawaii, January 22-24, 1992, in Honolulu.

Miller, Jeff. "The First Language," *UCSF Magazine* 13 (3): 31-33 (February 1992).

Morris, Robert. "Caring for the Family Facing Cancer." *Christian Ministry* 14(2): (March 1983) in Honolulu.

Nouwen, Henri J. M. *The Wounded Healer.* Garden City, N.Y.: Doubleday and Co., Inc., 1972.

Oates, Wayne E. *The Revelation of God in Human Suffering.* Philadelphia: Westminster Press, 1959.

Oden, Thomas C. *Pastoral Theology: Essentials of Ministry.* San Francisco: Harper and Row, 1983.

Packo, John E. *Coping with Cancer.* Camp Hill, Pa.: Christian Publications, 1991.

Passanisi, Kathleen Keller. Lecture given as part of the Value of Life symposium, Research Medical Center, Kansas City, May 6, 1993.

Pennington, Chester A. *Even So . . . Believe.* Nashville: Abingdon Press, 1966.

Purkiser, W. T., Richard S. Taylor, and Willard H. Taylor. *God, Man, and Salvation: A Biblical Theology.* Kansas City: Beacon Hill Press of Kansas City, 1977.

Swank, Grant J. "The Ministry of Being There." *The Preacher's Magazine* 68 (March, April, May 1992): 14.

Tengbom, Mildred. "Letting Tears Bring Healing and Renewal." *Care Notes,* St. Meinrad, Ind.: Abbey Press, 1990.

Walker, Alan. *How Jesus Helped People.* New York: Abingdon Press, 1964.

"What It Is That I Have, Don't Want, Didn't Ask For, Can't Give Back, and How I Feel About It." Columbus, Ohio: Ohio State University Comprehensive Cancer Center, Leukemia Society of America.

Wiersbe, Warren W. *Why Us? When Bad Things Happen to God's People.* Old Tappan, N.J.: Fleming H. Revell Co., 1984.

Wynkoop, Mildred Bangs. *A Theology of Love.* Kansas City: Beacon Hill Press of Kansas City, 1972.